INTRODUCTION

Definition of Intermittent Fasting

Intermittent fasting is a dietary approach that has gained widespread popularity in recent years. It involves alternating periods of eating and fasting, with the primary goal of regulating calorie intake and optimizing metabolic processes. The key feature of intermittent fasting is the cycling between periods of eating, known as "feeding windows," and periods of fasting, during which no or minimal calories are consumed.

Types of Intermittent Fasting

Intermittent fasting comes in various forms, each with its own unique approach. Some of the most common types include:

1. **16/8 Method**: This method involves fasting for 16 hours each day and limiting your eating to an 8-hour window. For example, you might eat between 12:00 PM and 8:00 PM and fast from 8:00 PM to 12:00 PM the next day.

2. **5:2 Diet**: In this approach, you consume your regular diet for five days of the week and drastically reduce calorie intake (around 500-600 calories) on the remaining two non-consecutive days.

3. **Eat-Stop-Eat**: This method includes fasting for a

full 24 hours once or twice a week. It typically involves fasting from dinner one day until dinner the next day.

4. **Alternate-Day Fasting**: This approach alternates between fasting days and regular eating days. On fasting days, calorie consumption is minimal or zero.

5. **The Warrior Diet**: This method consists of fasting for 20 hours and then having a 4-hour eating window in the evening. During the fasting period, small amounts of raw fruits and vegetables may be consumed.

How Intermittent Fasting Works

Intermittent fasting works on the principle of manipulating the body's insulin levels and metabolic processes. When you eat, especially carbohydrates, your body releases insulin to help transport glucose into cells for energy. Excessive insulin secretion can lead to weight gain and insulin resistance over time.

During fasting periods, insulin levels drop, and the body switches to burning stored fat for energy, a process known as ketosis. This fat-burning state can promote weight loss and other health benefits.

Benefits of Intermittent Fasting for Women Above 50

Intermittent fasting can be particularly advantageous for women above the age of 50. As women age, hormonal changes and a slower metabolism can make it more challenging to maintain a healthy weight and overall well-being. Here are some specific benefits of intermittent fasting for this demographic:

1. Weight Management

One of the primary benefits of intermittent fasting for women above 50 is its effectiveness in weight management. As metabolism naturally slows down with age, it becomes easier to gain weight. Intermittent fasting can help control calorie intake and promote fat loss, making it a valuable tool for maintaining a healthy weight.

2. Hormonal Balance

Hormonal fluctuations during menopause can lead to weight gain, mood swings, and other discomforts. Intermittent fasting may help regulate hormones, including insulin, which can contribute to more stable energy levels and mood.

3. Improved Insulin Sensitivity

Age-related insulin resistance can increase the risk of type 2 diabetes and weight gain. Intermittent fasting can enhance insulin sensitivity, allowing the body to utilize glucose more efficiently and potentially reduce the risk of diabetes.

4. Enhanced Cognitive Function

Intermittent fasting has been linked to improved brain health and cognitive function. For women above 50, this can be particularly beneficial in maintaining mental clarity and reducing the risk of cognitive decline.

5. Cardiovascular Health

Heart health becomes increasingly important with age. Intermittent fasting may improve various cardiovascular risk factors, such as blood pressure, cholesterol levels, and triglycerides, reducing the risk of heart disease.

6. Longevity

Studies in animals have suggested that intermittent fasting may extend lifespan by promoting cellular repair and reducing the risk of age-related diseases. While more research is needed in humans, this potential longevity benefit is intriguing.

7. Simplified Eating Patterns

For some women above 50, simplifying meal planning and timing through intermittent fasting can make it easier to maintain a healthy diet and lifestyle.

Purpose of the eBook

The purpose of this eBook is to provide comprehensive guidance and insights into the world of intermittent fasting, with a specific focus on its benefits for women above 50. This eBook aims to be a valuable resource for those who want to explore the concept of intermittent fasting, understand its principles, and harness its advantages for their health and well-being.

What the eBook Covers

This eBook will cover a wide range of topics related to intermittent fasting, including:

1. **Understanding Intermittent Fasting**: A detailed explanation of what intermittent fasting is, its various methods, and how it works.

2. **Benefits for Women Above 50**: Extensive information on how intermittent fasting can be particularly advantageous for women in this age group, addressing their unique health concerns.

3. **Getting Started**: Practical tips and step-by-step guidance on how to begin an intermittent fasting regimen safely and effectively.

4. **Meal Plans and Recipes**: Sample meal plans and nutritious recipes tailored to the needs of women above 50, making it easier to incorporate intermittent fasting into their daily lives.

5. **Common Questions and Concerns**: Answers to frequently asked questions and solutions to common challenges that may arise during intermittent fasting.

6. **Health and Safety**: A discussion on the importance of consulting with a healthcare professional before starting any new dietary regimen, especially for individuals with underlying health conditions.

7. **Success Stories**: Inspirational stories of women who have successfully incorporated intermittent fasting into their lives and reaped its benefits.

8. **Additional Resources**: References to further reading, research studies, and reputable sources for readers who want to delve deeper into the science and practice of intermittent fasting.

CHAPTER ONE

Understanding Intermittent Fasting

Different Types of Intermittent Fasting

Intermittent fasting (IF) has gained significant popularity in recent years due to its potential health benefits and effectiveness for weight management. There are various methods of intermittent fasting, each with its own unique approach. In this article, we will explore four popular types of intermittent fasting: the 16/8 Method, the 5:2 Method, the Eat-Stop-Eat Method, and the Alternate-Day Fasting Method.

The 16/8 Method

The 16/8 Method, also known as the Leangains protocol, is one of the most commonly practiced forms of intermittent fasting. It involves fasting for 16 hours each day and restricting your eating to an 8-hour window. For example, you might fast from 8:00 PM to 12:00 PM the next day, then eat your meals between 12:00 PM and 8:00 PM.

The main appeal of the 16/8 Method is its simplicity. It doesn't require drastic changes in your diet, making it easier to incorporate into your daily routine. During the fasting period, it's essential to stay hydrated and consume non-caloric beverages like water, herbal tea, or black coffee to help curb hunger.

One of the key benefits of this method is improved insulin

sensitivity, which can aid in better blood sugar control. Additionally, it may assist in weight loss by reducing daily calorie intake through a shortened eating window.

The 5:2 Method

The 5:2 Method involves eating normally for five days of the week and drastically reducing calorie intake for the remaining two days. On the fasting days, individuals typically consume around 500-600 calories. These fasting days are often referred to as "low-calorie" days.

For example, you might eat normally from Monday to Friday and then limit your calorie intake to 500-600 calories on Saturday and Sunday. This method allows for flexibility in choosing which days to fast, making it adaptable to individual schedules and preferences.

The 5:2 Method is believed to promote weight loss, improve metabolic health, and potentially enhance longevity. However, it's essential to plan your low-calorie days carefully, ensuring that you still receive essential nutrients during those periods.

The Eat-Stop-Eat Method

The Eat-Stop-Eat Method involves fasting for a full 24 hours once or twice a week. This means that you refrain from consuming any calories for an entire day. For example, you might finish dinner at 7:00 PM one day and then fast until 7:00 PM the following day.

This approach can be more challenging than some other intermittent fasting methods due to the extended fasting period. It requires discipline and careful consideration of your daily activities and energy levels during the fasting days. It's essential to stay hydrated during this fasting period.

The Eat-Stop-Eat Method is believed to promote significant calorie reduction, which can lead to weight loss over time. It also gives your digestive system a break and may support autophagy, a cellular process that removes damaged components, potentially benefiting overall health.

The Alternate-Day Fasting Method

Alternate-Day Fasting involves alternating between fasting days and regular eating days. On fasting days, you either abstain from food entirely or consume a very minimal amount of calories, usually around 500-600 calories. On non-fasting days, you can eat normally without restrictions.

For example, you might fast on Monday, eat as usual on Tuesday, fast again on Wednesday, and so on. This pattern continues throughout the week.

This method offers the potential for significant calorie reduction and weight loss, similar to the Eat-Stop-Eat Method. It can also improve insulin sensitivity and may have positive effects on heart health. However, it may not be suitable for everyone, as the fasting days can be challenging for some individuals to adhere to in the long term.

How Intermittent Fasting Works

Intermittent fasting works by altering the timing of when you eat, which can have various effects on your body's metabolism and hormonal balance. Here's a breakdown of how intermittent fasting operates:

1. **Insulin Sensitivity**: During fasting periods, insulin levels drop significantly. This allows your cells to become more sensitive to insulin when you do eat. Improved insulin sensitivity can help

regulate blood sugar levels and reduce the risk of type 2 diabetes.

2. **Fat Burning**: When you fast, your body enters a state of ketosis, where it starts burning stored fat for energy instead of relying on incoming food. This can lead to effective weight loss over time.

3. **Cellular Repair**: Fasting triggers a process called autophagy, where your cells remove damaged components and recycle them. This cellular repair mechanism may contribute to improved overall health and longevity.

4. **Hormone Regulation**: Fasting can affect the secretion of various hormones, such as growth hormone and norepinephrine, which play roles in fat burning and muscle preservation.

5. **Appetite Control**: Some people find that intermittent fasting helps them better control their appetite and reduce overall calorie intake, making it easier to maintain a healthy weight.

6. **Simplicity and Sustainability**: Intermittent fasting is relatively simple to implement and can be sustained in the long term. It doesn't require complex meal planning or counting calories, making it a practical approach for many individuals.

Safety Considerations

While intermittent fasting can offer numerous health benefits, it may not be suitable for everyone. Here are some safety considerations to keep in mind:

1. **Individual Variability**: People respond differently

to fasting, and what works well for one person may not be suitable for another. It's essential to listen to your body and consult with a healthcare professional before starting any fasting regimen, especially if you have underlying health conditions.

2. **Nutrient Intake**: During fasting periods, it's crucial to ensure you still receive essential nutrients. Make wise food choices on eating days to maintain a balanced diet. Consider consulting a registered dietitian for guidance.

3. **Dehydration**: Extended fasting periods can lead to dehydration. Stay hydrated by drinking water, herbal tea, or other non-caloric beverages during fasting periods.

4. **Energy Levels**: Some individuals may experience low energy levels, dizziness, or irritability while fasting. It's important to be mindful of these symptoms and adjust your fasting plan if necessary.

5. **Eating Disorders**: Intermittent fasting may not be suitable for individuals with a history of eating disorders or those prone to developing disordered eating patterns. If you have concerns about your relationship with food, consult with a mental health professional.

6. **Pregnancy and Nursing**: Pregnant or nursing women should avoid strict forms of intermittent fasting, as it may not provide adequate nutrition for the mother and baby.

CHAPTER TWO

Health Benefits

Weight Management

Weight management is a complex and multifaceted topic that encompasses various aspects of our health and well-being. It's not just about shedding excess pounds but also about achieving a balanced and sustainable lifestyle. Effective weight management involves a combination of healthy eating, regular physical activity, and mindful living.

Dietary Choices: One of the fundamental aspects of weight management is making mindful dietary choices. This includes consuming a balanced diet rich in whole grains, lean proteins, fruits, and vegetables. Avoiding processed foods high in sugars and unhealthy fats is crucial. Additionally, portion control plays a vital role in managing calorie intake.

Physical Activity: Regular exercise is indispensable for weight management. Engaging in a mix of aerobic exercises (like jogging or swimming) and strength training (such as weightlifting) can help increase metabolism, build muscle, and burn calories. Finding an exercise routine that you enjoy makes it easier to stay consistent.

Caloric Balance: Maintaining a healthy weight is largely about balancing the number of calories consumed with the number of calories expended. To lose weight, you need to create a calorie deficit by either eating fewer calories or increasing physical activity. Conversely, to gain weight, you need to consume more calories than you burn.

Mindful Eating: Mindful eating is a practice that involves paying close attention to your food, savoring each bite, and eating slowly. This approach can help you better understand your body's hunger and fullness cues, preventing overeating and promoting better weight management.

Emotional Well-being: Emotional factors can significantly impact weight management. Stress, anxiety, and depression can lead to emotional eating and cravings for comfort foods. Developing healthy coping mechanisms and seeking support when needed is crucial for emotional well-being and effective weight management.

Sleep: Adequate sleep is often underestimated in its role in weight management. Poor sleep can disrupt hormonal balance, increasing cravings for high-calorie foods and making it harder to control weight. Prioritizing a consistent sleep schedule is essential.

Long-Term Sustainability: Ultimately, the key to successful weight management is adopting sustainable lifestyle changes. Quick-fix diets and extreme exercise regimens are rarely effective in the long run. Instead, focus on gradual, sustainable changes that you can maintain over time.

In summary, weight management is not just about losing or gaining pounds but about achieving overall health and well-being through a combination of healthy eating, regular exercise, and mindful living.

Improved Metabolism

Metabolism is the body's complex system of chemical processes that convert food into energy and support various bodily functions. A well-functioning metabolism is essential for overall health and can have a significant impact on your energy levels and body composition.

Basal Metabolic Rate (BMR): Your BMR is the number of calories your body needs to maintain basic functions like breathing and circulation at rest. Factors like age, gender, and genetics influence your BMR. While you can't change these factors, you can boost your metabolism by increasing muscle mass through strength training.

Diet and Metabolism: What you eat directly affects your metabolism. Eating small, balanced meals throughout the day can help keep your metabolism active. Additionally, certain foods, such as spicy foods and those high in protein, may temporarily increase metabolism due to the thermic effect of food (TEF).

Physical Activity: Regular physical activity, particularly high-intensity interval training (HIIT) and strength training, can significantly enhance metabolism. These activities not only burn calories during the exercise but also increase the post-exercise calorie burn as your body repairs and builds muscle.

Hydration: Staying adequately hydrated is essential for efficient metabolism. Water is involved in many metabolic processes, and even mild dehydration can slow down your metabolism. Aim to drink enough water throughout the day.

Sleep and Stress: Lack of sleep and chronic stress can disrupt hormonal balance, negatively impacting metabolism. Prioritizing sleep and adopting stress-reduction strategies, such as meditation or yoga, can help maintain a healthy metabolism.

Thyroid Health: The thyroid gland plays a critical role in metabolism by producing hormones that regulate energy production. Thyroid disorders can lead to metabolic issues. If you suspect thyroid problems, consult a healthcare professional for evaluation and treatment.

Aging and Metabolism: Metabolism tends to slow down with age, primarily due to a loss of muscle mass. However, this natural process can be counteracted through regular physical activity and a well-balanced diet.

Mental Clarity and Focus

Mental clarity and focus are essential for productivity, decision-making, and overall cognitive well-being. Achieving and maintaining mental sharpness requires a combination of lifestyle choices and cognitive training.

Nutrition and Brain Health: A balanced diet rich in nutrients, especially omega-3 fatty acids, antioxidants, and B vitamins, can support brain health. These nutrients are found in foods like fatty fish, fruits, vegetables, and whole grains.

Hydration: Dehydration can impair cognitive function, leading to reduced focus and clarity. Ensure you drink enough water throughout the day to stay mentally sharp.

Sleep Quality: Quality sleep is crucial for cognitive function. During deep sleep, the brain consolidates memories and processes information. Aim for 7-9 hours of quality sleep each night to enhance mental clarity.

Stress Management: Chronic stress can fog the mind and hinder focus. Incorporate stress-reduction techniques like meditation, deep breathing exercises, or yoga into your daily routine to keep stress levels in check.

Regular Exercise: Physical activity increases blood flow to the brain, delivering oxygen and nutrients that support cognitive function. Incorporate regular aerobic exercise into your routine to boost mental clarity.

Mental Stimulation: Engaging in activities that challenge your brain, such as puzzles, reading, or learning a new skill, can help maintain mental clarity and focus.

Mindfulness and Meditation: Mindfulness practices and meditation can improve attention span and reduce mind-wandering, enhancing overall focus and clarity.

Limit Distractions: Minimize distractions in your environment, both digital and physical, to maintain focus during tasks that require concentration.

Heart Health

Maintaining a healthy heart is crucial for overall well-being. Your heart is responsible for pumping oxygen-rich blood throughout your body, supporting all vital organs and functions. Here are some key aspects of heart health:

Dietary Choices: A heart-healthy diet is rich in fruits, vegetables, whole grains, lean proteins, and healthy fats (such as those found in avocados and nuts). Limiting saturated and trans fats, as well as excessive sodium, is important to prevent heart disease.

Physical Activity: Regular exercise strengthens the heart muscle, improves circulation, and helps maintain a healthy weight. Aim for at least 150 minutes of moderate-intensity aerobic activity or 75 minutes of vigorous-intensity aerobic activity per week.

Blood Pressure Management: High blood pressure is a significant risk factor for heart disease. Monitoring and managing your blood pressure through lifestyle changes and medication, if necessary, is crucial.

Cholesterol Levels: High levels of LDL cholesterol ("bad" cholesterol) can contribute to plaque buildup in the arteries. Maintain healthy cholesterol levels through diet, exercise, and medication if prescribed by a healthcare professional.

Stress Reduction: Chronic stress can negatively impact heart health. Incorporate stress-reduction techniques such as meditation, deep breathing exercises, and yoga into your routine.

Smoking Cessation: Smoking is a major risk factor for heart disease. Quitting smoking is one of the most effective steps you can take to improve heart health.

Limit Alcohol: Excessive alcohol consumption can raise blood pressure and contribute to heart problems. If you choose to drink alcohol, do so in moderation.

Regular Check-ups: Schedule regular check-ups with your healthcare provider to assess your heart health, monitor risk factors, and make necessary adjustments to your lifestyle or medication.

Family History: If you have a family history of heart disease, be aware of your increased risk and take proactive steps to maintain heart health.

In conclusion, maintaining heart health involves a combination of dietary choices, regular physical activity, blood pressure and cholesterol management, stress reduction, avoiding smoking, limiting alcohol intake, regular check-ups, and awareness of family history. Prioritizing these aspects of heart health can significantly reduce the risk of cardiovascular disease.

Blood Sugar Control

Blood sugar control is essential for overall health, as imbalances can lead to various health issues, including diabetes. Here are key factors in managing blood sugar levels:

Balanced Diet: Consuming a balanced diet that includes complex carbohydrates, fiber, lean proteins, and healthy fats can help stabilize blood sugar levels. Avoid excessive consumption of refined sugars and high-glycemic foods.

Portion Control: Monitoring portion sizes can prevent overeating and help regulate blood sugar. Pay attention to portion sizes, especially when consuming carbohydrates.

Regular Meals: Eating regular meals and snacks throughout the day can help maintain steady blood sugar levels. Skipping meals can lead to blood sugar spikes and crashes.

Physical Activity: Exercise improves insulin sensitivity and helps regulate blood sugar. Aim for at least 150 minutes of moderate-intensity aerobic activity per week.

Medication and Insulin: If prescribed by a healthcare provider, take medications or insulin as directed to manage blood sugar levels.

Stress Management: Chronic stress can raise blood sugar

levels. Incorporate stress-reduction techniques such as meditation, yoga, or deep breathing exercises into your daily routine.

Monitor Blood Sugar: Regularly check your blood sugar levels as advised by your healthcare provider to track your progress and make necessary adjustments to your management plan.

Stay Hydrated: Proper hydration supports overall health, including blood sugar control. Drink enough water throughout the day.

Sleep: Quality sleep is essential for blood sugar regulation. Aim for 7-9 hours of sleep per night to support healthy blood sugar levels.

Cellular Autophagy

Cellular autophagy is a fascinating and essential process within our cells that plays a critical role in maintaining cellular health and preventing the buildup of damaged components. Autophagy is essentially a cellular "cleanup" mechanism that removes old, damaged organelles and proteins. Here's a closer look at this topic:

Definition: Autophagy, derived from Greek words meaning "self-eating," is a highly regulated process by which cells break down and recycle their damaged or dysfunctional components. It helps ensure cellular quality control and contributes to overall cell health.

Mechanism: Autophagy involves the formation of double-membraned structures called autophagosomes, which envelop and sequester cellular components to be degraded. These autophagosomes then fuse with lysosomes, where the cellular material is broken down and its components are recycled.

Benefits: Cellular autophagy has numerous benefits, including the removal of damaged organelles and proteins, clearance of harmful pathogens, and the recycling of cellular building blocks for energy production and cellular repair.

Induction of Autophagy: Several factors can induce autophagy, including nutrient deprivation, exercise, and certain dietary components. Intermittent fasting, for example, has been shown to stimulate autophagy, promoting cellular health.

Dysregulation and Disease: Dysfunctional autophagy has been implicated in various diseases, including neurodegenerative disorders like Alzheimer's and Parkinson's disease, cancer, and metabolic conditions. Maintaining healthy autophagy is crucial for preventing these diseases.

Promoting Autophagy: Strategies to promote autophagy include regular physical activity, a diet rich in antioxidants, and maintaining a healthy weight. Caloric restriction and intermittent fasting can also activate autophagy.

Aging and Autophagy: Autophagy tends to decline with age, contributing to the accumulation of cellular damage. Strategies that enhance autophagy, such as exercise and certain dietary patterns, may play a role in extending healthy lifespan.

In summary, cellular autophagy is a vital process that helps maintain cellular health by removing damaged components and recycling cellular materials. It can be promoted through lifestyle choices, including diet and exercise, and is implicated in various aspects of health and disease prevention.

Hormone Regulation

Hormones are chemical messengers produced by glands in the endocrine system. They play a central role in regulating various bodily functions, including metabolism, growth, mood, and reproductive processes. Achieving and maintaining hormone balance is essential for overall health and well-being.

Hormonal Imbalance: Hormonal imbalances can lead to a wide range of health issues. Common signs of hormonal imbalance include fatigue, mood swings, weight gain or loss, irregular menstrual cycles, and changes in skin and hair health.

Endocrine Glands: The endocrine system includes glands such as the pituitary, thyroid, adrenal, and pancreas. Each gland produces specific hormones that regulate different functions in the body.

Diet and Hormones: Nutrition plays a significant role in hormone regulation. Consuming a balanced diet that includes essential nutrients like vitamins, minerals, and healthy fats supports hormonal health. For example, omega-3 fatty acids are crucial for brain health and mood regulation.

Stress and Hormones: Chronic stress can disrupt hormone balance, leading to elevated levels of cortisol, the body's primary stress hormone. Practices like mindfulness, meditation, and adequate sleep can help manage stress and support hormone regulation.

Exercise and Hormones: Regular physical activity can help regulate hormones, including insulin and growth hormone. Exercise also promotes the release of endorphins, which improve mood and reduce stress.

Hormone Replacement Therapy: In cases of severe hormonal imbalance, hormone replacement therapy (HRT) may be recommended by healthcare professionals to restore hormone levels to a healthy range.

Age and Hormones: Hormone levels naturally fluctuate with age. For example, women experience menopause, which involves a decline in estrogen and progesterone levels. Hormone replacement therapy can alleviate some symptoms associated with menopause.

Consult a Healthcare Provider: If you suspect a hormonal imbalance, it's essential to consult a healthcare provider. They can perform tests to assess hormone levels and recommend appropriate treatment or lifestyle changes.

In conclusion, hormone regulation is crucial for overall health and involves maintaining balance through proper nutrition, stress management, regular exercise, and, when necessary, medical intervention. Hormones play a profound role in numerous bodily functions, and maintaining their balance is essential for well-being.

Longevity

Longevity refers to the length of an individual's lifespan. While genetics play a significant role in determining how long we live, lifestyle choices and environmental factors also have a substantial impact on our life expectancy. Here are some key factors related to longevity:

Genetics: Genetics plays a substantial role in determining our predisposition to certain diseases and our overall longevity. However, lifestyle choices can modulate genetic factors.

Healthy Diet: Consuming a balanced and nutritious diet is crucial for longevity. A diet rich in fruits, vegetables, whole grains, lean proteins, and healthy fats can reduce the risk of chronic diseases and promote longevity.

Physical Activity: Regular exercise is associated with a longer lifespan. It helps maintain a healthy weight, strengthens the cardiovascular system, and reduces the risk of conditions like heart disease and diabetes.

Stress Management: Chronic stress can have detrimental effects on health and longevity. Effective stress management techniques, such as meditation, yoga, and spending time in nature, can help increase life expectancy.

Social Connections: Maintaining strong social connections and a sense of community has been linked to increased longevity. Social engagement provides emotional support and a sense of belonging.

Avoiding Smoking and Excessive Alcohol: Smoking and excessive alcohol consumption are significant risk factors for premature death. Quitting smoking and moderating alcohol intake can have a positive impact on longevity.

Preventive Healthcare: Regular check-ups and screenings can help detect and address health issues early, improving the chances of successful treatment and longevity.

Quality Sleep: Quality sleep is essential for overall health and longevity. Aim for 7-9 hours of restorative sleep each night.

Mindfulness: Practices like mindfulness meditation can promote emotional well-being and may contribute to a longer, healthier life

CHAPTER THREE

Getting Started

Setting Realistic Goals

Setting realistic goals is a crucial step in achieving success, whether it's in your personal life or professional endeavors. Unrealistic goals can lead to frustration and disappointment, while realistic ones provide motivation and a sense of accomplishment. Here, we'll delve into the importance of setting realistic goals and provide some practical tips to help you get started.

Why Set Realistic Goals?

1. Avoiding Overwhelm: One of the primary reasons to set realistic goals is to avoid overwhelm. When you set goals that are too ambitious or far-fetched, you might find yourself overwhelmed with the sheer magnitude of what you're trying to achieve. This can lead to stress and burnout.

2. Sustaining Motivation: Realistic goals are attainable, and as you make progress towards them, you'll experience a sense of accomplishment. This positive reinforcement can boost your motivation and keep you on track.

3. Measurable Progress: Realistic goals can be measured, which allows you to track your progress effectively. You can see how far you've come and make adjustments as needed.

Tips for Setting Realistic Goals

1. Define Clear Objectives: Start by clearly defining what you want to achieve. Whether it's related to your career, health, or personal development, having a specific goal in mind is essential.

2. Break It Down: Divide your larger goal into smaller, more manageable tasks or milestones. This makes the process less daunting and gives you a sense of direction.

3. Consider Resources and Constraints: Take into account the resources you have available and any constraints you might face. Realistic goals should be aligned with what's feasible given your circumstances.

4. Be Time-Bound: Set a timeline for achieving your goals. This helps create a sense of urgency and prevents procrastination.

5. Prioritize and Focus: It's essential to prioritize your goals. Trying to tackle too many things at once can dilute your efforts. Focus on one or two key goals at a time.

Preparing Your Kitchen

Preparing your kitchen is a fundamental step in adopting a healthier lifestyle and making better food choices. A well-organized kitchen can streamline meal preparation, encourage nutritious eating, and save you time and money. Let's explore how to set up your kitchen for success.

Organizing Your Kitchen

1. Declutter: Start by decluttering your kitchen. Remove any items that are expired or rarely used. A clutter-free kitchen is more pleasant to work in.

2. Stock Essentials: Ensure you have essential ingredients on hand, such as whole grains, lean proteins, fruits, and vegetables. Having these items readily available makes it easier to prepare balanced meals.

3. Invest in Kitchen Tools: Consider investing in quality kitchen tools like a sharp chef's knife, cutting boards, and cookware. Having the right tools can make cooking more efficient and enjoyable.

Creating a Healthy Environment

1. Visibility Matters: Keep healthy foods, like fruits and veggies, visible and within easy reach. Place them at eye level in your fridge and pantry, so they're the first things you see.

2. Minimize Junk Food: If possible, reduce the presence of unhealthy snacks and sugary drinks in your kitchen. If they're not readily available, you're less likely to indulge in them.

3. Meal Prep Zone: Dedicate an area of your kitchen as a meal prep zone. This can be a countertop space where you can chop vegetables, assemble meals, and portion out snacks.

Creating a Meal Plan

Meal planning is a powerful tool for maintaining a balanced diet and staying on track with your nutrition goals. It helps you make informed food choices, reduce food waste, and save time. Here's how to create an effective meal plan.

Steps to Create a Meal Plan

1. Set Your Goals: Start by defining your dietary goals. Are you aiming to lose weight, gain muscle, or simply eat healthier? Your goals will influence your meal plan.

2. Choose Nutrient-Rich Foods: Base your meals on nutrient-rich foods like vegetables, lean proteins, whole grains, and healthy fats. These foods provide essential nutrients without excess calories.

3. Plan Your Meals: Decide how many meals and snacks you'll have each day. Then, plan the specific meals, considering variety and balance.

4. Portion Control: Pay attention to portion sizes to avoid overeating. Using measuring cups and a food scale can help with accurate portioning.

5. Make a Shopping List: Once your meals are planned, create a shopping list. Stick to the list when you go grocery shopping to avoid impulse purchases.

6. Prep in Advance: Spend some time each week preparing ingredients or entire meals in advance. This can save you time during busy weekdays.

Tracking Progress

Tracking your progress is essential to ensure you're moving in the right direction and to stay motivated on your journey. Whether it's related to your health and fitness goals or personal development, here's how to effectively track your progress.

Tools for Tracking Progress

1. Journals and Notebooks: Keeping a journal or notebook allows you to record your daily or weekly progress. You can jot down achievements, setbacks, and insights.

2. Apps and Technology: Many apps and digital tools are designed for tracking various goals, such as fitness, nutrition, and habit-building. They can provide valuable data and insights.

3. Visual Aids: Create visual aids like charts, graphs, or vision boards to represent your progress visually. This can be especially motivating as you see your accomplishments accumulate.

Setting Milestones

1. Short-Term and Long-Term Goals: Break your larger goal into smaller milestones. Short-term goals should be achievable within a few weeks or months, while long-term goals may take several months or even years.

2. Celebrate Achievements: When you reach a milestone, celebrate your achievements. Acknowledging your progress can boost your motivation to keep going.

3. Adjust as Needed: Regularly review your progress and be open to making adjustments to your goals or strategies if necessary. Sometimes, circumstances change, and flexibility is key to success.

CHAPTER FOUR

Intermittent Fasting Protocols

The 16/8 Protocol

The 16/8 fasting protocol, also known as the time-restricted eating method, has gained popularity as a simple and effective way to improve metabolic health and aid in weight management. This approach involves fasting for 16 hours and restricting your eating to an 8-hour window within a 24-hour day.

Daily Schedule

The daily schedule for the 16/8 protocol typically begins with a fasting period that lasts from the evening until the following morning. Here's a sample daily schedule:

- **6:00 AM:** Wake up and start your day.
- **10:00 AM:** Begin your 8-hour eating window.
- **2:00 PM:** Enjoy your first meal.
- **6:00 PM:** Consume your last meal of the day.
- **8:00 PM:** Start your 16-hour fasting period.

During the fasting period, it's essential to stay hydrated by drinking water, herbal tea, or black coffee, as these beverages are allowed during fasting.

Sample Meal Plan

Creating a balanced meal plan during the 16/8 protocol is crucial to ensure you meet your nutritional needs while staying within the eating window. Here's a sample meal plan for this fasting method:

Breakfast (2:00 PM):

- Spinach and feta omelet
- Mixed berries

Lunch (4:00 PM):

- Grilled chicken breast
- Steamed broccoli
- Quinoa

Snack (6:00 PM):

- Greek yogurt with honey
- Almonds

Dinner (7:30 PM):

- Baked salmon
- Roasted asparagus
- Brown rice

Remember that the key to success with the 16/8 protocol is to prioritize nutrient-dense foods and avoid excessive calorie consumption during the eating window.

The 5:2 Protocol

The 5:2 fasting protocol, also known as the Fast Diet, gained popularity due to its flexibility. This method involves eating regularly for five days a week and significantly reducing calorie intake for the other two days, often referred to as "fasting days."

Explanation of the Method

The 5:2 protocol is based on intermittent fasting, and it allows for a caloric intake of around 500-600 calories on fasting days. These two fasting days are not required to be consecutive, giving you the flexibility to choose when they fit into your schedule. On non-fasting days, you can eat your regular diet without restrictions.

This approach may help with weight loss and offers potential health benefits like improved insulin sensitivity and reduced inflammation.

Sample Meal Plan

Here's a sample meal plan for one of the fasting days in the 5:2 protocol:

Fasting Day Meal Plan:

- Breakfast (10:00 AM):
    - Scrambled eggs with spinach
    - A small apple
- Lunch (1:00 PM):
    - Grilled vegetable salad with a light vinaigrette dressing
- Snack (4:00 PM):
    - A handful of carrot sticks with hummus
- Dinner (7:00 PM):
    - Baked cod fish
    - Steamed broccoli
    - A small portion of quinoa

It's crucial to maintain proper hydration on fasting days and consult with a healthcare professional before starting this or any fasting protocol, especially if you have underlying health conditions.

The Eat-Stop-Eat Protocol

The Eat-Stop-Eat protocol is an intermittent fasting method that involves full-day fasting once or twice a week. This approach was popularized by Brad Pilon in his book of the same name.

Explanation of the Method

During a full-day fast in the Eat-Stop-Eat protocol, you abstain from all calorie consumption for a 24-hour period. For example, if you start your fast at dinner one day, you wouldn't eat again until dinner the next day. This fasting method can be done once or twice a week, depending on your goals and comfort level.

The extended fasting periods in Eat-Stop-Eat may lead to a significant calorie deficit, which can promote weight loss and improve insulin sensitivity. However, it's important to ensure that you stay adequately hydrated during fasting days.

Sample Meal Plan

Here's a sample meal plan for a non-fasting day in the Eat-Stop-Eat protocol:

Non-Fasting Day Meal Plan:

- Breakfast (8:00 AM):
    - Overnight oats with almond butter and berries
- Lunch (12:00 PM):
    - Grilled chicken salad with mixed greens and balsamic vinaigrette
- Snack (3:30 PM):
    - Celery sticks with peanut butter
- Dinner (7:00 PM):
    - Stir-fried tofu with vegetables and brown rice

Remember to adjust your meal plans accordingly on fasting days by abstaining from all food consumption and focusing on staying hydrated.

The Alternate-Day Fasting Protocol

Alternate-day fasting (ADF) is an intermittent fasting method that alternates between fasting days and regular eating days. It has gained attention for its potential benefits in terms of weight loss and metabolic health.

Explanation of the Method

In the Alternate-Day Fasting protocol, you alternate between days of fasting, where you consume very few calories or none at all, and days of regular eating. This pattern repeats itself throughout the week, allowing for flexibility in meal planning. Some people choose to consume a minimal amount of calories (around 500) on fasting days, while others may opt for complete fasting.

7 days Sample Meal Plan

Here's a sample 7-day meal plan to illustrate how the Alternate-Day Fasting protocol might work:

Day 1 (Fasting):
- **Fasting Day:** Consume only water, herbal tea, or black coffee.

Day 2 (Eating):
- **Breakfast (8:00 AM):**
  - Greek yogurt with honey and walnuts
- **Lunch (12:30 PM):**
  - Turkey and avocado wrap with whole-grain bread
- **Snack (3:00 PM):**
  - Sliced cucumbers with hummus

- **Dinner (7:00 PM):**
    - Grilled salmon with roasted sweet potatoes and green beans

Day 3 (Fasting):
- **Fasting Day:** Consume only water, herbal tea, or black coffee.

Day 4 (Eating):
- Repeat the meal plan from Day 2.

Continue alternating between fasting and eating days throughout the week. It's crucial to stay hydrated on fasting days and consult with a healthcare professional before adopting this or any fasting protocol.

Day 5 (Fasting):
- **Fasting Day:** Consume only water, herbal tea, or black coffee.

Day 6 (Eating):
- **Breakfast (8:00 AM):**
    - Scrambled eggs with spinach and tomatoes
- **Lunch (12:30 PM):**
    - Quinoa salad with chickpeas, cucumber, and a lemon-tahini dressing
- **Snack (3:00 PM):**
    - Sliced bell peppers with guacamole
- **Dinner (7:00 PM):**
    - Grilled chicken breast with roasted Brussels sprouts and brown rice

Day 7 (Fasting):
- **Fasting Day:** Consume only water, herbal tea, or black coffee.

CHAPTER FIVE

Tips and Tricks

Staying Hydrated

Staying hydrated is essential for overall health and well-being. It's a topic that often seems straightforward, but there are nuances to consider. Proper hydration affects various aspects of your life, from physical performance to cognitive function.

Importance of Hydration

Hydration is not just about drinking water. It's about maintaining a delicate balance of fluids in your body. Water is vital for digestion, circulation, absorption of nutrients, and the regulation of body temperature. Without adequate hydration, you may experience fatigue, dizziness, and even more severe health issues like kidney stones.

The 8x8 rule is a common guideline. This suggests drinking eight 8-ounce glasses of water per day. However, individual water needs vary based on factors like age, activity level, and climate. You might need more or less than this guideline suggests.

Signs of Dehydration

Recognizing dehydration is crucial. Some common signs include dark urine, dry mouth, dizziness, and reduced urine output. However, thirst is not always a reliable indicator, especially in older adults. It's important to listen to your body and ensure you're drinking enough fluids regularly.

Dehydration can affect your mental clarity. Even mild dehydration can lead to cognitive deficits, including reduced concentration and alertness. To stay mentally sharp, keeping well-hydrated is essential.

Tips for Staying Hydrated

Incorporate water-rich foods. Fruits and vegetables like watermelon, cucumber, and oranges have high water content and can contribute to your daily hydration needs.

Carry a reusable water bottle. Having a water bottle with you can serve as a visual reminder to drink throughout the day.

Set hydration goals. Challenge yourself to drink a certain amount of water by specific times of the day. This can help ensure you meet your hydration needs.

Managing Hunger

Hunger is a natural sensation that our bodies use to signal the need for nourishment. However, managing hunger effectively can be challenging, especially in a world filled with tempting but unhealthy food options.

Understanding Hunger

Hunger comes in different forms. There's physical hunger, which is a genuine need for sustenance, and emotional hunger, which stems from stress, boredom, or other emotional triggers. It's essential to differentiate between the two to make informed choices.

Hunger is regulated by hormones. Ghrelin is the hormone responsible for signaling hunger, while leptin signals fullness. These hormones can be influenced by factors such as sleep, stress, and meal timing.

Strategies for Managing Hunger

Eat balanced meals. Meals that include a combination of protein, fiber, and healthy fats can help you feel fuller for longer. This reduces the likelihood of snacking between meals.

Stay hydrated. Sometimes, thirst is mistaken for hunger. Before reaching for a snack, drink a glass of water and see if your hunger subsides.

Mindful eating can help. Pay attention to your body's hunger cues and eat slowly. This allows your brain to register fullness, preventing overeating.

Incorporating Exercise

Exercise is a crucial component of a healthy lifestyle. It not only helps maintain physical fitness but also has numerous mental and emotional benefits.

Types of Exercise

Exercise comes in various forms. Cardiovascular exercises like running and cycling improve cardiovascular health, while strength training builds muscle mass and bone density. Flexibility exercises like yoga enhance mobility.

Combining different types of exercise is ideal. A balanced fitness routine should include a mix of cardiovascular, strength, and flexibility exercises to target different aspects of your health.

Benefits of Regular Exercise

Physical benefits are extensive. Regular exercise can improve cardiovascular health, increase muscle tone, and boost metabolism. It's also a powerful tool for weight management.

Exercise has mental health benefits. It releases endorphins, which are natural mood lifters. Regular exercise can help reduce stress, anxiety, and symptoms of depression.

Tips for Incorporating Exercise

Find activities you enjoy. Whether it's dancing, hiking, or playing a sport, choose activities that you find fun. This increases the likelihood of sticking to a regular exercise routine.

Set realistic goals. Gradually build up your exercise routine to avoid burnout and injury. Start with manageable goals and progress from there.

Schedule exercise like an appointment. Treat exercise as a non-negotiable part of your day. This helps establish a consistent routine.

Dealing with Social Situations

Navigating social situations can be challenging when you're trying to maintain a healthy lifestyle. Whether it's peer pressure to eat unhealthy foods or feeling uncomfortable at social gatherings, these situations can test your commitment.

Social Pressure

Peer pressure is real. It's common to feel pressured to indulge in unhealthy foods or drinks in social settings. It's essential to stay true to your goals and make choices that align with your health priorities.

Communication is key. If you're comfortable, explain your goals to your friends and loved ones. They may be more understanding and supportive than you think.

Healthy Socializing

Look for healthier options. When dining out or attending parties, seek out nutritious choices on the menu or bring a healthy dish to share.

Focus on the social aspect, not just the food. Remember that social gatherings are about connecting with others. Engage in conversations and activities to divert your attention from unhealthy temptations.

Overcoming Plateaus

Plateaus are frustrating but common in any journey toward better health. Whether you're trying to lose weight or improve your fitness, hitting a plateau can be discouraging. However, it's important to remember that plateaus are not permanent.

Plateau Causes

Plateaus can occur due to various reasons. Your body may have adapted to your current workout routine or diet, leading to a lack of progress. Stress, inadequate sleep, and hormonal changes can also contribute.

Stress the importance of patience. Plateaus are a natural part of the process. It's crucial to stay patient and not get discouraged.

Strategies for Breaking Plateaus

Change your routine. If you've been doing the same exercises or eating the same foods for a while, it might be time to switch things up. Try new workouts or modify your diet.

Track your progress. Keeping a journal of your workouts, meals, and how you feel can help identify patterns and areas for improvement.

Seek professional guidance. If you're struggling to break a plateau, consider consulting a fitness trainer or nutritionist who can provide personalized advice.

CHAPTER SIX

Common Mistakes to Avoid

Overeating During Eating Windows

Overeating during eating windows is a common issue that many people face, especially when they are following intermittent fasting or time-restricted eating patterns. The concept of eating windows restricts the hours during which individuals can consume their meals, which can sometimes lead to overindulgence. This behavior can have adverse effects on one's health and overall well-being.

Understanding Eating Windows: Eating windows are specific time frames during the day when individuals are allowed to eat their meals. For example, an individual might have an eating window from 12:00 PM to 8:00 PM. During this time, they can consume their meals, but outside of this window, only water, tea, or other non-caloric beverages are allowed. This approach is often used as a tool for weight management and improving metabolic health.

The Pitfall of Overeating: One of the common pitfalls of eating windows is the temptation to overeat within the allowed time frame. People might feel that they need to consume all their daily calories within this limited window, leading to larger portion sizes and potentially unhealthy food choices. This can negate the benefits of intermittent fasting and may result in weight gain rather than loss.

Strategies to Avoid Overeating: To prevent overeating during eating windows, it's essential to practice mindful eating. This means being aware of hunger and fullness cues and listening to your body's needs. Additionally, you can plan balanced and nutritious meals to ensure that you're getting the necessary nutrients without overindulging. Portion control is also crucial; using smaller plates and utensils can help you manage portion sizes effectively.

The Importance of Balanced Nutrition: Another key aspect is to focus on the quality of the food you consume during your eating window. Opt for whole foods like fruits, vegetables, lean proteins, and whole grains. Avoid excessive consumption of processed and high-calorie foods, as they can lead to overeating and provide little nutritional value.

In summary, while eating windows can be a useful tool for managing calorie intake and improving metabolic health, it's crucial to be mindful of overeating within these time frames. Practicing mindful eating, portion control, and prioritizing nutrient-dense foods can help individuals make the most of their eating windows without falling into the trap of overindulgence.

Ignoring Hydration

Hydration is a fundamental aspect of maintaining good health, yet many people tend to ignore their body's need for adequate water intake. Ignoring hydration can lead to various health issues and can impact one's daily life in significant ways.

The Importance of Hydration: Water is essential for the proper functioning of the human body. It plays a vital role in digestion, circulation, temperature regulation, and overall cellular function. When the body is not adequately hydrated, it can lead to problems such as fatigue, dizziness, dry skin, constipation, and even more severe conditions like kidney stones or heatstroke.

Common Reasons for Ignoring Hydration: Several factors contribute to individuals ignoring their hydration needs. One of the most common reasons is simply forgetting to drink water throughout the day. Busy schedules, distractions, and lack of awareness can all contribute to this oversight. Additionally, some people may intentionally limit their water intake to reduce bathroom trips, which can disrupt their work or daily routine.

Health Consequences: Ignoring hydration can have several health consequences. Dehydration can lead to reduced cognitive function, making it challenging to focus and perform daily tasks efficiently. It can also affect physical performance during exercise, as muscles require adequate hydration to function optimally. Chronic dehydration can contribute to long-term health issues, including urinary tract infections and kidney problems.

Strategies for Staying Hydrated: To avoid the negative effects of ignoring hydration, it's essential to develop strategies to stay adequately hydrated. Some tips include carrying a reusable water bottle with you throughout the day, setting reminders to drink water, and tracking your daily water intake. Additionally, consuming water-rich foods like fruits and vegetables can contribute to your overall hydration.

In conclusion, ignoring hydration is a common but detrimental habit that can lead to various health issues. Recognizing the importance of staying hydrated and implementing strategies to meet your daily water needs is essential for maintaining good health and well-being.

Unrealistic Expectations

Setting unrealistic expectations, whether in personal or professional life, can lead to disappointment, stress, and a sense of failure. It's crucial to strike a balance between ambition and realism to achieve one's goals effectively.

The Nature of Unrealistic Expectations: Unrealistic expectations are beliefs or goals that are set too high and are often unattainable within a reasonable timeframe or with available resources. These expectations can relate to career achievements, relationships, personal development, or even physical appearance. They often stem from societal pressure, comparison with others, or a lack of understanding of one's own capabilities.

The Consequences of Unrealistic Expectations: When individuals set unrealistic expectations, they may experience several negative consequences. First and foremost is the feeling of constant disappointment when goals are not met. This can lead to low self-esteem, anxiety, and depression. Unrealistic expectations can also strain relationships, as individuals may project their unmet goals onto others or become overly demanding.

Strategies for Managing Expectations: Managing expectations effectively is essential for maintaining mental and emotional well-being. Here are some strategies to consider:

1. **Self-awareness:** Reflect on your own abilities and limitations. Understand that everyone has strengths and weaknesses, and it's okay not to excel in everything.

2. **Set realistic goals:** Break down larger goals

into smaller, achievable steps. This can make daunting tasks more manageable and increase the likelihood of success.

3. **Seek support:** Talk to friends, family, or a therapist about your expectations and concerns. They can provide valuable perspectives and emotional support.

4. **Practice gratitude:** Focus on what you have accomplished rather than what you haven't. Cultivating a sense of gratitude can improve overall happiness.

5. **Adjust as needed:** It's okay to reassess and adjust your expectations as circumstances change. Flexibility is a valuable trait in adapting to life's challenges.

Skipping Regular Check-ups

Regular check-ups with healthcare professionals are crucial for monitoring one's health and detecting potential issues early. However, many people tend to skip these appointments for various reasons, which can have serious consequences for their well-being.

The Importance of Regular Check-ups: Regular check-ups, such as annual physical exams and dental visits, are essential for preventive healthcare. These appointments allow healthcare providers to assess a person's overall health, screen for diseases, and provide early interventions if necessary. Detecting health problems in their early stages often leads to more effective treatments and better outcomes.

Common Reasons for Skipping Check-ups: Several factors contribute to individuals skipping regular check-ups:

1. **Fear or Anxiety:** Some people have a fear of medical procedures or bad news, which makes them avoid healthcare appointments.

2. **Busy Lifestyle:** Busy schedules can make it challenging to prioritize health check-ups, especially when there are no apparent symptoms.

3. **Cost:** Healthcare costs can be a barrier, particularly for those without insurance or with high deductibles.

4. **Denial:** Some individuals may deny the importance of regular check-ups, believing that they are healthy and do not need them.

Health Consequences: Skipping regular check-ups can lead to delayed diagnosis and treatment of health conditions. Conditions that could have been managed or cured in their early stages may progress to more advanced and challenging-to-treat stages. This can lead to worsened health outcomes and, in some cases, increased healthcare costs in the long run.

Strategies for Prioritizing Check-ups: To ensure that regular check-ups are not skipped, consider the following strategies:

1. **Schedule in Advance:** Plan your check-ups well in advance, and make them a part of your annual calendar.

2. **Find a Trusted Healthcare Provider:** Establish a relationship with a healthcare provider you trust and feel comfortable with.

3. **Understand the Importance:** Educate yourself about the benefits of preventive healthcare and

early detection of health issues.

4. **Financial Planning:** If cost is a concern, research options for affordable healthcare or inquire about payment plans with your provider.

5. **Overcoming Fear:** If fear or anxiety is a barrier, consider talking to a mental health professional to address these issues.

CHAPTER SEVEN

Success Stories

Real-life Testimonials

Real-life testimonials are powerful tools that can help businesses build trust and credibility with their potential customers. These testimonials are essentially statements or reviews from real people who have used a product or service and are willing to share their experiences. In the world of marketing and advertising, they serve as social proof, reassuring potential customers that they are making a wise choice. Let's explore the significance of real-life testimonials and how they can impact consumers' decision-making processes.

The Power of Authenticity

Authenticity is key when it comes to real-life testimonials. In a world where consumers are bombarded with advertisements and sales pitches, they are becoming increasingly discerning. Authentic testimonials resonate with people because they are relatable. When potential customers read or hear about the experiences of others who have faced similar challenges or needs, they are more likely to trust the product or service being endorsed.

These testimonials should feel real and unscripted. Authenticity can be further emphasized by using the actual words of the person giving the testimonial.

Quotes that sound too polished or rehearsed may raise suspicions among consumers. Businesses should encourage customers to share their honest opinions, even if they include constructive criticism.

Building Trust and Credibility

One of the primary functions of real-life testimonials is to **build trust and credibility**. When consumers see that others have had positive experiences with a product or service, they are more likely to believe that they will too. Trust is a crucial factor in purchasing decisions, especially for products or services that involve a significant investment or have a long-term impact.

Businesses can highlight the credentials or backgrounds of the individuals giving the testimonials to enhance credibility. For example, if a renowned chef endorses a brand of cookware, it carries more weight than an endorsement from an unknown individual. However, both can be effective, as long as they come across as genuine.

Emotional Connection

Real-life testimonials often evoke **emotional responses** from potential customers. When people read or hear about the positive changes a product or service has brought into someone's life, they can imagine experiencing those changes themselves. Emotional connection can be a powerful motivator in the decision-making process.

To maximize the emotional impact of testimonials, businesses should encourage customers to share their personal stories. Whether it's a heartwarming tale of how a fitness program helped someone regain their health or a story about a skincare product boosting someone's confidence, these narratives can resonate deeply with others who share similar aspirations.

Overcoming Objections

One of the main obstacles in the buyer's journey is overcoming objections or doubts. Real-life testimonials can **address common objections** in a persuasive manner. If potential customers have concerns about a product's effectiveness, cost, or ease of use, testimonials can provide real-world examples of how those concerns were successfully addressed.

For instance, if a software company receives feedback that some users find their product too complicated, they can feature a testimonial from a customer who initially felt the same way but eventually found the software user-friendly after some guidance and practice. This can be a powerful way to alleviate concerns and encourage hesitant buyers to take action.

Diversity in Testimonials

To reach a broader audience and increase the impact of testimonials, it's important to **feature a diverse range of voices and experiences**. Different people have different needs and preferences, and potential customers are more likely to find testimonials compelling if they can relate to the individuals giving them. This diversity can encompass factors such as age, gender, ethnicity, and background.

For example, a skincare brand can showcase testimonials from individuals with various skin types and concerns. This shows potential customers that the product is versatile and suitable for a wide range of people. It also demonstrates inclusivity and makes customers feel that the brand values and represents diversity.

In conclusion, real-life testimonials are potent tools in

marketing and advertising. They provide authenticity, build trust and credibility, create emotional connections, address objections, and appeal to a diverse audience. Businesses should prioritize collecting and showcasing these testimonials to help potential customers make informed and confident purchasing decisions.

CHAPTER EIGHT

Frequently Asked Questions

Addressing Common Queries

In the world of customer service and information dissemination, addressing common queries effectively is a paramount task. It involves not only providing answers but also ensuring that those answers are clear, concise, and easily accessible to your audience. In this discussion, we will delve into various strategies and best practices for addressing common queries in a manner that leaves your audience satisfied and well-informed.

Understanding the Importance of Addressing Queries

Addressing common queries is more than just a customer service routine; it's an essential aspect of maintaining a positive relationship with your audience. Here are a few reasons why addressing queries effectively matters:

1. **Customer Satisfaction**: Timely and accurate responses to common queries greatly enhance customer satisfaction. When customers feel heard and valued, they are more likely to remain loyal to your brand.

2. **Reduced Workload**: By addressing common queries efficiently, you can reduce the workload on your customer support team, freeing them up to focus on more complex issues.

3. **Building Trust**: Providing accurate and helpful information builds trust with your audience. Trust is a fundamental component of a successful business relationship.

4. **Enhanced Brand Reputation**: Brands that consistently provide clear and helpful responses to common queries earn a positive reputation in the eyes of consumers.

Strategies for Addressing Common Queries

Now that we understand the importance of addressing common queries, let's explore some effective strategies for doing so:

1. Create a Comprehensive FAQ Section

One of the most straightforward ways to address common queries is by creating a comprehensive FAQ (Frequently Asked Questions) section on your website or platform. Here's how to do it effectively:

- **Identify Common Questions**: Start by identifying the most frequently asked questions related to your products or services.
- **Organize by Categories**: Organize the questions into categories to make navigation easier for users.
- **Clear and Concise Answers**: Provide clear, concise, and jargon-free answers to each question.
- **Regular Updates**: Keep the FAQ section up-to-date. As new questions arise, add them to the list.

2. Implement Chatbots and AI-Powered Tools

Chatbots and AI-powered tools can significantly streamline the process of addressing common queries. Here's how:

- **24/7 Availability**: Chatbots can provide instant responses round the clock, ensuring that customers get answers when they need them.

- **Data Analysis**: AI tools can analyze customer queries to identify trends and update your FAQ section accordingly.

- **Personalization**: Chatbots can provide personalized responses based on user data, enhancing the customer experience.

3. Encourage User-Generated Content

User-generated content, such as forums and discussion boards, can be valuable for addressing common queries. Here's how to leverage it effectively:

- **Moderation**: Ensure that the user-generated content is moderated to maintain a respectful and informative environment.

- **Recognition**: Acknowledge and reward users who provide helpful answers to common queries.

- **Integration**: Integrate user-generated content with your official FAQ section for a holistic approach.

4. Proactive Communication

Sometimes, addressing queries proactively can prevent them from becoming common queries. Here's how to do it:

- **Email Updates**: Send regular email updates to your customers, highlighting new features, changes, and potential issues they should be aware of.

- **Video Tutorials**: Create video tutorials or webinars to educate your audience on using your products or services effectively.

- **Surveys and Feedback**: Collect feedback from your customers and use it to preemptively address potential concerns.

5. Provide Multiple Contact Channels

Not all customers prefer the same communication channel. Offering multiple options can enhance the way you address common queries:

- **Live Chat**: Implement live chat support for real-time responses.
- **Email**: Offer email support for more detailed inquiries.
- **Phone Support**: Provide a phone hotline for customers who prefer voice communication.
- **Social Media**: Monitor and respond to queries on social media platforms.

The Art of Crafting Clear Responses

Addressing common queries effectively also hinges on how well you craft your responses. Here are some tips for ensuring clarity and effectiveness in your answers:

1. Use Plain Language

Avoid jargon and technical terms unless your audience is well-versed in them. Use plain language that anyone can understand.

2. Keep It Concise

While it's essential to provide thorough answers, avoid unnecessary verbosity. Get to the point quickly to maintain the reader's interest.

3. Use Visual Aids

Wherever applicable, use visual aids such as diagrams, screenshots, or infographics to supplement your explanations.

4. Link to Additional Resources

If a query requires an in-depth explanation, provide links to relevant articles, guides, or videos for those who want to explore the topic further.

5. Be Empathetic

Show empathy towards the user's query or concern. Acknowledge their issue and assure them that you're there to help.

Handling Difficult Queries

Not all queries are easy to address, and some may involve complex or sensitive issues. Here's how to handle them effectively:

1. Escalation Protocols

Establish clear escalation protocols for queries that cannot be resolved through standard channels. Ensure that customers know how to escalate their concerns.

2. Transparent Communication

If a query involves a problem or mistake on your end, be transparent about it. Apologize if necessary and explain the steps you're taking to rectify the situation.

3. Empower Your Support Team

Provide your support team with the necessary training and resources to handle difficult queries professionally and empathetically.

4. Learn from Feedback

Collect feedback from customers who had difficult queries. Use this feedback to improve your processes and prevent similar issues in the future.

Conclusion

Recap of Benefits

In a world filled with endless choices and opportunities, people often seek clarity and reassurance before making decisions. This is where a recap of benefits becomes a valuable tool, helping individuals understand the advantages of a particular product, service, or course of action. In this discussion, we will delve into the significance of recapping benefits and explore how it can empower individuals to make informed choices.

Why Recap Benefits?

Recapping benefits serves several essential purposes:

1. **Clarity**: It provides clarity by summarizing the key advantages of a product or service. This clarity helps individuals grasp the value proposition quickly.

2. **Reinforcement**: It reinforces the positive aspects of a choice, reminding individuals why they considered it in the first place. This reinforcement is crucial for maintaining enthusiasm.

3. **Comparison**: It allows for easy comparison between options, making it simpler for individuals to weigh the pros and cons of each.

4. **Decision-Making**: It aids in decision-making. When faced with multiple options, a recap of benefits can be the deciding factor in choosing one over the others.

How to Effectively Recap Benefits

To be effective, a recap of benefits should follow some key

principles:

1. Highlight the Most Relevant Benefits

Not all benefits are created equal. Some are more important to the target audience than others. Start by identifying the benefits that resonate the most with your audience, and ensure these are prominently featured in the recap.

2. Use Clear and Concise Language

Avoid jargon and complex language. Use simple, clear, and concise language that anyone can understand. The goal is to make the benefits easily digestible.

3. Visual Aids

Incorporate visual aids like charts, graphs, or infographics to present data and statistics. Visuals can significantly enhance the impact of your benefit recap.

4. Tell a Story

Craft a narrative around the benefits. People are more likely to remember a story than a list of facts. Share real-life examples or testimonials that illustrate how the benefits have positively impacted others.

5. Address Concerns

Acknowledge potential concerns or objections that your audience might have. Then, explain how the benefits address these concerns. This demonstrates empathy and builds trust.

6. Create a Sense of Urgency

Encourage action by emphasizing why it's important to act now rather than later. Limited-time offers, exclusive bonuses, or impending deadlines can create a sense of urgency.

Examples of Effective Benefit Recaps

1. Fitness App Subscription

Imagine you're marketing a fitness app subscription. An effective benefit recap might look like this:

- **Benefit 1**: Achieve Your Dream Body - Get in shape and feel confident.
- **Benefit 2**: Convenience at Your Fingertips - Work out anytime, anywhere.
- **Benefit 3**: Expert Guidance - Access to certified trainers for personalized workouts.
- **Benefit 4**: Track Your Progress - Monitor your fitness journey and celebrate milestones.
- **Benefit 5**: Community Support - Connect with like-minded individuals for motivation.

This recap emphasizes the core benefits that resonate with fitness enthusiasts: physical transformation, accessibility, expert guidance, progress tracking, and community support.

2. Online Learning Platform

If you're promoting an online learning platform, your benefit recap might look like this:

- **Benefit 1**: Expand Your Knowledge - Access a vast library of courses on diverse subjects.
- **Benefit 2**: Flexible Learning - Study at your own pace and on your schedule.
- **Benefit 3**: Expert Instructors - Learn from industry professionals and experts.
- **Benefit 4**: Career Advancement - Acquire new skills to boost your career.
- **Benefit 5**: Interactive Learning - Engage with quizzes, assignments, and discussions.

This recap highlights the advantages of flexible, expert-led learning for personal and professional growth.

Encouragement and Motivation

Encouragement and motivation are powerful driving forces in human life. They play a crucial role in helping individuals overcome challenges, reach their goals, and achieve personal growth. In this section, we will explore the significance of encouragement and motivation and how they can positively impact individuals.

The Power of Encouragement

Encouragement is a form of support that provides individuals with the confidence and belief that they can succeed. It serves as a boost to one's self-esteem and can significantly impact their willingness to take risks and face challenges. Here are some key aspects of the power of encouragement:

1. Boosting Confidence

When someone believes in us and encourages our efforts, it boosts our confidence. This increased self-assurance can be a game-changer, enabling us to tackle tasks that might have seemed daunting otherwise.

2. Fostering Resilience

Encouragement helps build resilience. It teaches individuals that setbacks are not failures but opportunities to learn and grow. This mindset shift is crucial for long-term success.

3. Strengthening Relationships

Offering encouragement can strengthen relationships, whether in personal or professional settings. It creates a positive and supportive atmosphere where individuals feel valued and appreciated.

4. Fueling Determination

Encouragement fuels determination. When people feel encouraged, they are more likely to persist in their efforts and push through obstacles.

The Essence of Motivation

Motivation is the inner drive that compels individuals to take action toward their goals. It's the fuel that keeps us moving forward, even when faced with challenges. Here are some fundamental aspects of motivation:

1. Intrinsic vs. Extrinsic Motivation

Motivation can be either intrinsic (coming from within) or extrinsic (externally driven). Intrinsic motivation, such as pursuing a hobby out of passion, is often more sustainable and fulfilling in the long run.

2. Setting Clear Goals

Motivation thrives when there are clear, achievable goals in sight. Setting specific objectives provides a sense of purpose and direction.

3. Overcoming Procrastination

Motivation can help individuals overcome procrastination. When the desire to achieve a goal is strong, it becomes easier to prioritize tasks and manage time effectively.

4. Adapting to Challenges

Motivation enables individuals to adapt to challenges. It fuels problem-solving and encourages the exploration of creative solutions.

Practical Strategies for Encouragement and Motivation

Encouragement and motivation are not just abstract concepts; they can be cultivated and applied in various aspects of life. Here are some practical strategies for both giving and receiving encouragement and motivation:

Giving Encouragement:

1. **Be Specific**: When offering encouragement, be specific about what you admire or appreciate in the individual. General praise is less impactful than targeted compliments.

2. **Active Listening**: Listen actively when someone shares their goals or challenges. Show empathy and offer support tailored to their needs.

3. **Set Realistic Expectations**: Encourage realistic goals and expectations. Unrealistic goals can lead to disappointment and demotivation.

4. **Celebrate Progress**: Acknowledge and celebrate small wins along the way. Celebrating milestones provides a sense of achievement.

Receiving Motivation:

1. **Visualize Success**: Visualize yourself achieving your goals. This mental imagery can boost motivation and focus.

2. **Seek Accountability**: Share your goals with someone who can hold you accountable. This external support can be a powerful motivator.

3. **Break Tasks Down**: Divide larger tasks into smaller, manageable steps. Achieving these mini-goals can boost motivation and reduce overwhelm.

4. **Stay Inspired**: Surround yourself with sources

of inspiration, whether it's quotes, books, or mentors. Continuous inspiration can fuel motivation.

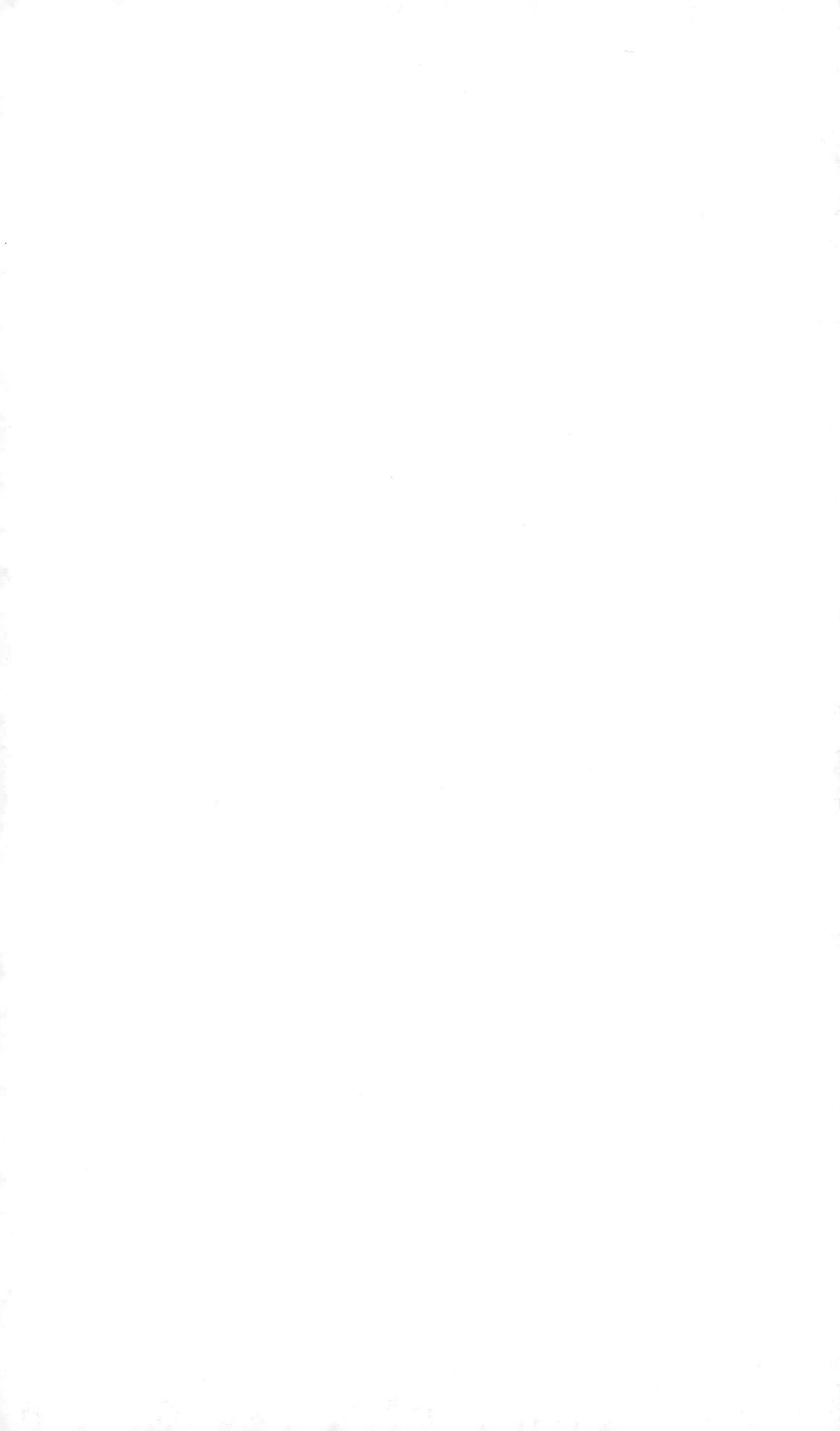